Living With Parkinson's Disease

Unshaken: Embracing Life with Parkinson's

BY

Dr. Luna Jefferson

Copyright

TABLE OF CONTENT

Introduction to Parkinson's Disease

Parkinson's disease is a complex and pervasive neurological disorder that impacts millions of lives worldwide. Named after the physician who first described its symptoms in 1817, Dr. James Parkinson, this condition has been the subject of extensive research and continues to pose a significant challenge to individuals, families, and the medical community.

At its core, Parkinson's disease is characterized by the gradual loss of dopamine-producing neurons in a specific region of the brain called the substantia nigra. Dopamine is a neurotransmitter responsible for transmitting signals that control movement and coordination. As these neurons degenerate, it leads to a disruption in the brain's communication pathways, resulting in the hallmark motor symptoms of Parkinson's, such as tremors, bradykinesia (slowness of movement), and muscle rigidity.

But Parkinson's is not merely a motor disorder; it can also affect various aspects of a person's life, including their mood, cognition, and even their sense of smell. Additionally, the causes of Parkinson's remain a subject of ongoing research, with factors ranging from genetics to environmental exposures being examined.

This introduction is just the beginning of our journey into the world of Parkinson's disease. We will delve deeper into its causes, symptoms, diagnosis, treatments, and the resilient individuals who navigate life with this condition. Understanding Parkinson's is the first step towards empowerment and improved quality of life for those living with the disease and their loved ones.

Historical Viewpoint

The historic point of view of Parkinson's disease is a demonstration of the getting through journey for information and human compasion notwithstanding testing clinical secrets. The foundations of understanding this condition can be followed back to old human advancements. It was the old Indian text, the "Rigveda," that previously portrayed a condition looking like the quakes of Parkinson's.

In any case, it was only after the early 19th century that the condition earned respect as an unmistakable clinical substance.

In 1817, English doctor Dr. James Parkinson distributed "An Article on the Shaking Paralysis," where he illustrated the clinical highlights of the infection that would later bear his name. Dr. Parkinson's work was significant in revealing insight into the condition and featuring its crippling impacts.

Throughout the long term, clinical science has taken significant steps in figuring out the pathology and reasons for Parkinson's illness. This has considered more exact finding and treatment systems. During the twentieth 100 years, the disclosure that the deficiency of dopamine-creating neurons assumed a focal part in Parkinson's additionally developed our understanding of the disease.

Today, with continuous examination and innovative advances, our verifiable viewpoint has developed into a powerful scene of logical investigation, pushing us closer to opening the secrets of Parkinson's disease. The excursion from old works to present day nervous system science is a demonstration of the tirelessness of the clinical local area and the enduring obligation to mitigating the experiencing brought about by this complex neurological problem.

The Significance of Parkinson's Disease

Parkinson's disease carries profound significance not only in the realm of healthcare but in the lives of those it touches. Beyond its medical dimensions, the significance of Parkinson's disease extends to society, caregivers, and the global healthcare landscape.

First and foremost, Parkinson's is a significant medical challenge. It ranks among the most prevalent neurodegenerative disorders, affecting millions of individuals worldwide. Its hallmark motor symptoms, including tremors, slowness of movement, and muscle rigidity, can profoundly impact one's ability to carry out everyday tasks and maintain independence. Non-motor symptoms, such as cognitive decline and mood changes, further complicate the clinical picture.

The significance of Parkinson's also reverberates through families and caregivers. The burden on those caring for individuals with Parkinson's can be emotionally, physically, and financially demanding. The importance of support systems and resources for both patients and caregivers cannot be overstated. Moreover, in the broader context, Parkinson's disease underscores the pressing need for research into neurodegenerative disorders. It serves as a reminder of the urgency in understanding the intricate workings of the brain and developing treatments for these devastating conditions. Advances in Parkinson's research often have ripple effects, benefitting the broader field of neuroscience and other neurodegenerative diseases.

In conclusion, the significance of Parkinson's disease is multi-faceted, encompassing the medical, personal, societal, and research realms. It stands as a poignant reminder of the challenges faced by those with neurodegenerative conditions and the collective responsibility to improve the lives of those affected.

CHAPTER ONE

What Is Parkinson's Disease?

Parkinson's disease, often referred to simply as Parkinson's, is a chronic and progressive neurological disorder that primarily affects movement. It takes its name from Dr. James Parkinson, who in 1817 published "An Essay on the Shaking Palsy," a seminal work that provided the first comprehensive description of the condition. Today, Parkinson's remains a complex and multifaceted disorder with far-reaching implications.

At its core, Parkinson's disease is characterized by the degeneration of dopamine-producing neurons in a specific region of the brain called the substantia nigra. Dopamine is a neurotransmitter responsible for transmitting signals that control movement and coordination. As these neurons gradually decline, the brain's ability to regulate and fine-tune motor functions is compromised.

The cardinal motor symptoms of Parkinson's disease include tremors (involuntary shaking), bradykinesia (slowness of movement), muscle rigidity, and postural instability, which can lead to balance problems and an increased risk of falls. However, Parkinson's is not solely a motor disorder; it often encompasses a wide array of non-motor symptoms, such as changes in speech, mood, and cognition, along with disturbances in sleep and autonomic functions.

Though the exact causes of Parkinson's disease are not yet fully understood, it is believed to involve a combination of genetic and environmental factors. Ongoing research seeks to uncover the intricate mechanisms underlying the disease and explore potential treatments to improve the lives of those affected. Parkinson's disease represents a significant challenge in the field of neurology and a poignant reminder of the need for continued research, care, and support for those living with this condition.

Anatomy of the Brain and Nervous System

The brain and nervous system are the body's most intricate and vital communication network, responsible for controlling every thought, sensation, and movement. Understanding their complex anatomy is fundamental to comprehending neurological conditions like Parkinson's disease.

The brain, encased in the skull, consists of several distinct regions, each with specific functions. The cerebral cortex, the outermost layer, is responsible for higher cognitive functions, including thinking, problem-solving, and conscious awareness. The basal ganglia, a group of structures deep within the brain, plays a critical role in regulating motor movements, and its dysfunction is closely linked to Parkinson's.

The spinal cord, an extension of the brain, carries signals to and from the brain and the rest of the body. Nerves branch out from the spinal cord to transmit electrical impulses throughout the body, enabling sensory perception and motor control. It's these intricate connections and pathways that allow us to perform daily activities, from walking to complex problem-solving.

In Parkinson's disease, the substantia nigra, a structure in the midbrain, is of particular significance. It's here that dopamine-producing neurons degenerate, leading to the hallmark motor symptoms of the condition. The disruption in dopamine signaling within the basal ganglia creates a cascade of movement-related challenges.

Appreciating the intricacies of the brain and nervous system is fundamental to understanding how Parkinson's disease disrupts this complex network and hinders the communication between the brain and the body. This insight is key to both diagnosis and the development of effective treatments for neurological conditions.

Basics of Dopamine

Dopamine is a pivotal neurotransmitter in the brain, with profound effects on various aspects of human life, from movement and mood to motivation and reward. Understanding the basics of dopamine is essential when exploring conditions like Parkinson's disease, which are intricately tied to dopamine's role in the brain.

Dopamine is produced in clusters of nerve cells, or neurons, primarily found in two regions of the brain: the substantia nigra and the ventral tegmental area (VTA). These neurons play a central role in regulating motor function, emotions, and the brain's reward system.

One of dopamine's primary functions is to facilitate communication between neurons. It acts as a chemical messenger, transmitting signals from one neuron to another across synapses, which are the tiny gaps between nerve cells. In the context of movement, dopamine helps regulate motor control by fine-tuning the brain's instructions to muscles.

The brain's reward system heavily relies on dopamine. It plays a key role in feelings of pleasure, motivation, and reinforcement, making it central to activities such as eating, exercise, and even addictive behaviors.

In Parkinson's disease, the most recognizable issue is the loss of dopamine-producing neurons in the substantia nigra. This deficiency leads to the hallmark motor symptoms of the disease, as the brain struggles to coordinate movements effectively.

Dopamine is not just a chemical; it is a fundamental driver of our actions, emotions, and experiences. Understanding its role in the brain is crucial not only for comprehending conditions like

Parkinson's but also for unlocking the mysteries of our complex neurological system.

The Role of the Substantia Nigra

The substantia nigra is a crucial structure nestled deep within the brain's midbrain. Its significance lies in its pivotal role in controlling movement and motor function. Understanding the function of the substantia nigra is essential in grasping the pathophysiology of conditions like Parkinson's disease.

The substantia nigra is primarily responsible for producing dopamine, a neurotransmitter that serves as a critical messenger in the brain's intricate network. Dopamine is essential for transmitting signals that regulate voluntary muscle movements. This region of the brain is divided into two parts: the pars compacta, which is responsible for dopamine production, and the pars reticulata, which helps regulate the flow of information within the basal ganglia.

In Parkinson's disease, the substantia nigra is profoundly affected. Dopamine-producing neurons in the pars compacta degenerate, resulting in a significant reduction in dopamine levels. This imbalance in dopamine signaling within the basal ganglia leads to motor dysfunction, causing the characteristic symptoms of the disease, including tremors, bradykinesia (slowness of movement), and muscle rigidity.

The substantia nigra's role in motor control is so critical that its dysfunction disrupts the brain's ability to coordinate movement effectively, ultimately impacting a person's ability to carry out even the simplest daily tasks.

Appreciating the central role of the substantia nigra in the brain's motor control system is fundamental in understanding how and why Parkinson's disease manifests and why treatments often focus on restoring dopamine levels or modulating dopamine signaling within this key region.

CHAPTER TWO

Unraveling the Mystery: Causes and Risk Factors

The causes and risk factors of Parkinson's disease have long been a subject of intense scientific investigation, yet much of the condition's origin remains shrouded in mystery. This complex neurological disorder is believed to arise from a combination of genetic and environmental factors, making it a puzzle that continues to challenge researchers and healthcare professionals. Genetics play a significant role in some cases of Parkinson's. Familial or inherited forms of the disease have been linked to specific genetic mutations, although these account for only a small percentage of cases. In most instances, Parkinson's is considered sporadic, with no clear hereditary component.

Nonetheless, genetic studies have shed light on potential risk factors and pathways involved in the disease.

Environmental factors also come into play. Exposure to toxins like pesticides, herbicides, and industrial chemicals has been associated with an increased risk of developing Parkinson's. Research has identified a potential link between rural living, well water consumption, and the disease, further underscoring the multifaceted nature of its causes.

Other factors such as age, sex, and lifestyle choices may contribute to the risk of Parkinson's. The disease is more prevalent in older individuals, and men are somewhat more likely to develop it than women. Smoking and caffeine consumption have shown some protective effects, while head injuries and a history of certain medical conditions may increase risk.

Despite decades of research, Parkinson's disease's precise origins remain elusive. The interplay of genetic and environmental factors continues to be explored, offering hope that unlocking this mystery will lead to better prevention and treatment strategies for this challenging condition.

Genetic Factors in Parkinson's Disease

Genetic factors play a notable role in understanding the origins of Parkinson's disease. While the majority of cases are sporadic and not directly inherited, there are several genes associated with familial or hereditary forms of the condition. These genetic insights have provided valuable clues into the complex nature of Parkinson's.

Mutations in certain genes have been linked to familial Parkinson's disease. The most well-known of these is the SNCA gene, which encodes for alpha-synuclein, a protein that accumulates in the brains of Parkinson's patients. Mutations in the LRRK2, PINK1, and Parkin genes have also been identified, each contributing to specific forms of hereditary Parkinson's. Additionally, variations in the GBA gene are associated with an increased risk of Parkinson's disease. This gene is involved in the metabolism of lipids and the accumulation of abnormal proteins in the brain, both of which are hallmarks of the condition.

While these genetic factors provide important insights, they account for a relatively small proportion of all Parkinson's cases. Most individuals with Parkinson's do not have a known family history of the disease, and their condition is believed to result from a complex interplay of genetic and environmental factors. Understanding the genetic factors associated with Parkinson's disease is a significant step forward in unraveling the condition's mysteries. It not only aids in identifying those at higher risk but also informs ongoing research aimed at developing targeted therapies and interventions. Ultimately, the complex genetic landscape of Parkinson's underscores the need for a multifaceted approach in addressing this challenging neurological disorder.

Environmental Triggers in Parkinson's Disease

While genetic factors play a crucial role in the development of Parkinson's disease, environmental triggers also come into play, potentially contributing to the risk of this neurological disorder. Environmental factors can vary widely, but some have been extensively studied in relation to Parkinson's disease.

1. Pesticides and Herbicides: Exposure to certain chemicals used in agriculture and landscaping has been linked to an increased risk of Parkinson's. Pesticides like paraquat and organophosphates have garnered particular attention. These substances can disrupt the brain's dopamine-producing cells, contributing to the disease's progression.

2. Industrial Toxins: Some industrial chemicals, such as solvents and heavy metals (e.g., lead and manganese), have been associated with a higher risk of Parkinson's. These toxins can accumulate in the brain, leading to neurodegeneration.

3. Well Water Contamination: Some studies have suggested that consuming well water with high levels of certain minerals, like iron or manganese, may be a risk factor for Parkinson's. The source of the well water, geographic location, and specific minerals present can all play a role.

4. Head Injuries: Traumatic brain injuries, especially repeated concussions or severe head injuries, may increase the risk of developing Parkinson's disease later in life.

5. Living in Rural Areas: Studies have shown a higher incidence of Parkinson's in rural areas, although the reasons for this association are still under investigation. It is believed to involve factors such as well water, pesticide exposure, and lifestyle differences.

6. Viruses and Infections: Emerging research suggests that certain viral infections and inflammation may contribute to the development of Parkinson's disease, though the mechanisms involved are complex.

Understanding the environmental triggers of Parkinson's disease is essential in the quest to prevent and treat the condition effectively. Research in this area continues to expand, shedding light on the interplay between genetics and environmental factors, ultimately contributing to a more comprehensive understanding of this complex neurological disorder.

The Connection Between Genetics and Environment in Parkinson's Disease

Parkinson's disease is a prime example of the intricate interplay between genetics and the environment in the development of complex neurological disorders. While genetic factors and environmental triggers are often considered separately, they are inextricably linked in the pathogenesis of Parkinson's.

Genetics provides a foundation for understanding hereditary forms of the disease, where specific mutations in certain genes increase the risk. For instance, mutations in the SNCA, LRRK2, and Parkin genes have strong genetic ties to familial Parkinson's. However, these hereditary cases represent a minority of those affected by the disease.

For the majority of Parkinson's cases, environmental factors are believed to play a crucial role. Exposure to toxins like pesticides, herbicides, and industrial chemicals can lead to neurotoxic effects, particularly on dopamine-producing neurons. These environmental triggers can influence the risk of developing Parkinson's, even in individuals without a strong genetic predisposition.

The connection between genetics and the environment is further underscored by gene-environment interactions. Some genetic variants may increase vulnerability to environmental toxins, making individuals more susceptible to developing Parkinson's when exposed to certain triggers. Conversely, some genetic factors may provide protective effects, mitigating the impact of environmental risks.

Understanding the complex interplay between genetics and the environment in Parkinson's disease is vital for both research and clinical practice. It emphasizes the need for a personalized approach to diagnosis and treatment, where an individual's genetic profile and environmental history are considered to develop targeted therapies and interventions. This multifaceted perspective is key to unraveling the mysteries of Parkinson's disease and developing effective strategies for prevention and management.

CHAPTER THREE

Recognizing the Enemy: Signs and Symptoms of Parkinson's Disease

Parkinson's disease manifests through a constellation of signs and symptoms that significantly impact an individual's quality of life. Recognizing these clinical features is essential for early diagnosis and effective management of the condition.

1. Tremors: One of the most recognizable symptoms is resting tremors, typically starting in one hand or finger. These tremors often occur when the affected limb is at rest and decrease during purposeful movement.

2. Bradykinesia: Slowness of movement is a hallmark of Parkinson's. Everyday activities become challenging as patients experience a gradual loss of spontaneous movements and a delay in initiating actions.

3. Muscle Rigidity: Muscles become stiff and inflexible, leading to discomfort and sometimes pain. Rigidity affects the limbs and neck, contributing to difficulty in tasks like turning or bending.

4. Postural Instability: Parkinson's patients often struggle with balance and coordination, making them susceptible to falls. This postural instability can have serious consequences for their safety.

5. Changes in Gait: Walking patterns alter, resulting in shorter steps, shuffling, and difficulty with directional changes. Individuals may feel as though they're stuck to the ground.

6. Non-Motor Symptoms: Parkinson's is not limited to motor symptoms. It can affect cognitive function, mood, and autonomic functions, leading to problems like depression, anxiety, constipation, and sleep disturbances.

7. Hypomimia: Reduced facial expression, known as hypomimia, is another characteristic sign, making the face appear expressionless.

Understanding the full spectrum of Parkinson's symptoms is crucial for early detection and prompt intervention. While there's no cure for the disease, timely diagnosis and symptom management, often through medications and therapy, can significantly improve the quality of life for those living with Parkinson's. Furthermore, ongoing research aims to develop treatments that may slow or modify the disease's progression, providing hope for the future.

The Cardinal Symptoms of Parkinson's Disease

Parkinson's disease is characterized by a set of cardinal symptoms, often referred to as the "TRAP" acronym: Tremors, Rigidity, Akinesia (slowness of movement), and Postural Instability. These hallmark symptoms collectively define the clinical presentation of Parkinson's and are instrumental in its diagnosis.

1. Tremors: Resting tremors, typically starting on one side of the body, are a defining feature of Parkinson's disease. They manifest as rhythmic, involuntary shaking, most noticeable at rest and often abating during voluntary movement. Tremors usually begin in the hand or fingers, resembling the repetitive "pill-rolling" motion.

2. Rigidity: Muscle rigidity is another key symptom, leading to stiffness and inflexibility of the limbs and joints. It often results in a "cogwheel" or "lead-pipe" resistance to passive movement during physical examinations.

3. Akinesia: Akinesia, or slowness of movement, is characterized by a gradual loss of spontaneous and automatic movements. Simple actions, such as buttoning a shirt or walking, become slower and more deliberate.

4. Postural Instability: Postural instability refers to impaired balance and coordination, making individuals more prone to falls. It becomes particularly pronounced as the disease progresses, and maintaining a steady posture becomes challenging.

These cardinal symptoms represent the core clinical features of Parkinson's disease and are essential in its diagnosis. While non-motor symptoms and individual variations can complicate the clinical picture, identifying and addressing these core motor symptoms early on is crucial for the effective management and quality of life for those living with Parkinson's. Research and treatments continue to focus on these fundamental aspects of the disease in the quest to improve the lives of patients and their caregivers.

Lesser-Known Symptoms of Parkinson's Disease

Parkinson's disease is not just limited to the well-known motor symptoms; it often brings with it a spectrum of lesser-known, yet equally significant, non-motor symptoms. These less visible aspects of the disease can significantly affect a person's quality of life and should not be underestimated.

1. Cognitive Changes: While Parkinson's is primarily a movement disorder, it frequently presents with cognitive impairments. These can range from mild memory difficulties to more severe conditions like dementia. Individuals may experience challenges with attention, problem-solving, and executive functions.

2. Mood Disorders: Depression and anxiety are prevalent among those with Parkinson's. These emotional challenges can be as debilitating as the motor symptoms, often requiring specialized care and attention.

3. Sleep Disturbances: Sleep problems are common and can include insomnia, restless legs syndrome, and REM sleep behavior disorder. These disturbances can lead to excessive daytime sleepiness and a decrease in overall well-being.

4. Autonomic Dysfunction: Parkinson's can disrupt the autonomic nervous system, causing symptoms like constipation, urinary problems, and blood pressure fluctuations. These issues can significantly impact daily life.

5. Hyposmia: A reduced sense of smell, known as hyposmia, is frequently observed in Parkinson's disease. This symptom can

precede motor symptoms by several years and serves as a potential early indicator.

6. Pain: Pain is an often underreported symptom in Parkinson's. Musculoskeletal pain, dystonia-related pain, and off-period pain are among the discomforts that can occur.

7. Speech and Swallowing Difficulties: Changes in speech patterns, including reduced volume and clarity, and swallowing difficulties, can hinder effective communication and lead to potential health risks.

These lesser-known symptoms in Parkinson's disease highlight the complex and multisystem nature of the condition. A holistic approach to care that addresses both motor and non-motor aspects is essential for enhancing the overall well-being of individuals living with Parkinson's. Recognizing and managing these less visible challenges is vital for providing comprehensive and compassionate support to patients and their families.

The Stages of Parkinson's Disease

Parkinson's disease is a progressive neurodegenerative condition, and its progression is often divided into several stages. These stages provide a framework for understanding the evolving nature of the disease and its impact on an individual's life. It's important to note that not all individuals with Parkinson's will experience the same progression, and the rate at which the disease advances can vary significantly.

1. Early Stage: In the initial stages, individuals may experience mild motor symptoms, often affecting one side of the body. Tremors, bradykinesia (slowness of movement), and rigidity may be present but are typically manageable. Non-motor symptoms may also appear, such as mood changes and sleep disturbances.

2. Moderate Stage: As the disease progresses, motor symptoms become more pronounced and start to affect both sides of the body. Individuals may experience difficulties with daily tasks and mobility, leading to an increased risk of falls. Non-motor symptoms, including cognitive changes, may become more apparent.

3. Advanced Stage: In this stage, motor symptoms become severe and debilitating, making daily activities increasingly challenging. Individuals may have difficulty walking, experience significant rigidity, and face a higher risk of falls and injuries. Non-motor symptoms, including mood disorders and cognitive impairment, become more pronounced and may require specialized care.

4. Advanced Complications: In the most advanced stage, individuals often experience severe motor impairments, including freezing of gait and severe bradykinesia. They may become wheelchair-bound or bedridden, requiring extensive care. Non-motor complications, such as dysphagia (swallowing difficulties), are more common and necessitate significant support.

It's crucial to understand that these stages provide a general overview of the disease's progression. However, the experience of Parkinson's varies from person to person, and the timing and severity of symptoms can differ widely. Effective management and care in each stage can significantly improve an individual's quality of life, making early diagnosis and appropriate

intervention critical in the journey with Parkinson's.

CHAPTER FOUR

Diagnosis and Beyond in Parkinson's Disease

Diagnosing Parkinson's disease is a complex and often challenging process that involves a thorough medical evaluation, including a comprehensive clinical assessment, medical history, and neurological examinations. Beyond the diagnosis itself, the journey with Parkinson's involves ongoing care, management, and adaptation to the evolving nature of the condition.

Diagnosis: A Parkinson's diagnosis is primarily based on the presence of hallmark motor symptoms, including resting tremors, bradykinesia (slowness of movement), muscle rigidity, and postural instability. A neurologist may also consider the response to dopaminergic medication, a critical diagnostic criterion. However, there's no definitive test for Parkinson's, which can lead to misdiagnoses or delayed diagnoses.

Differential Diagnosis: Because the symptoms of Parkinson's can resemble other neurological conditions, differential diagnosis is crucial. Conditions like essential tremor, multiple system atrophy, and drug-induced parkinsonism can mimic Parkinson's, making it essential to rule out these possibilities.

Importance of Early Diagnosis: Early diagnosis is critical in Parkinson's disease, as it allows for more effective management and the potential to slow the progression of the disease. Medications, physical therapy, and lifestyle adjustments can help maintain quality of life in the early stages.

Ongoing Management: Beyond diagnosis, individuals living with Parkinson's require ongoing care and management. This often includes medication management to alleviate symptoms and improve function. Physical therapy, occupational therapy, and speech therapy can be essential in maintaining mobility and communication skills.

Coping and Support: Parkinson's is not just a physical challenge; it also brings emotional and psychological burdens. Coping with mood changes, cognitive impairments, and the progressive nature of the disease is part of the journey. Support from family, friends, and support groups can provide a vital lifeline for both patients and caregivers.

Parkinson's is a complex and evolving condition, and the journey doesn't end with diagnosis. A comprehensive, multidisciplinary approach to care and an understanding of the many dimensions of the disease are crucial in improving the lives of individuals living with Parkinson's.

The Diagnostic Process in Parkinson's Disease

Diagnosing Parkinson's disease is a complex and often time-consuming process that requires the expertise of a neurologist or movement disorder specialist. Since there's no single definitive test for Parkinson's, the diagnosis relies on a combination of clinical evaluation, medical history, and specialized assessments.

1. Clinical Assessment: The diagnostic journey typically begins with a thorough clinical evaluation. The neurologist or specialist will conduct a detailed interview to gather information about the patient's medical history, including any family history of neurological disorders or Parkinson's. They will also inquire about the patient's specific symptoms and how they have progressed over time.

2. Neurological Examination: A comprehensive neurological examination is fundamental to the diagnosis. The physician assesses the patient's motor functions, looking for hallmark signs of Parkinson's, including resting tremors, bradykinesia (slowness of movement), muscle rigidity, and postural instability.

3. Response to Medication: A key diagnostic criterion is the patient's response to dopaminergic medications, like levodopa. If there is a noticeable improvement in motor symptoms after taking these medications, it suggests a positive response, which is typical of Parkinson's.

4. Differential Diagnosis: Since other conditions can mimic Parkinson's disease, a critical aspect of the diagnostic process is excluding other potential causes. Conditions like essential tremor, multiple system atrophy, and drug-induced parkinsonism are among the differential diagnoses that must be considered.

5. Imaging Studies: In some cases, neuroimaging studies like MRI or DaTSCAN may be used to support the diagnosis. These tests can help rule out other conditions and provide additional insights into brain structures and function.

The diagnostic process in Parkinson's disease can be challenging due to its complexity and the absence of a single definitive test. It often involves multiple assessments and close collaboration between the patient, their healthcare team, and specialists to arrive at an accurate diagnosis. Early and accurate diagnosis is vital for initiating appropriate treatment and support, improving the patient's quality of life throughout the journey with Parkinson's.

Differential Diagnosis in Parkinson's Disease

Differential diagnosis is a critical aspect of evaluating and diagnosing Parkinson's disease, a condition that shares clinical features with other movement disorders and neurological conditions. It involves a systematic process of distinguishing between Parkinson's and similar disorders to arrive at an accurate diagnosis.

1. Essential Tremor: Essential tremor is a common movement disorder characterized by rhythmic, involuntary shaking of the hands and other body parts. While resting tremors are a hallmark of Parkinson's, essential tremor is typically seen during voluntary movements and may be misidentified as Parkinson's tremors.

2. Multiple System Atrophy (MSA): MSA is another neurodegenerative disorder that can mimic Parkinson's, as it often presents with similar motor symptoms. However, MSA

tends to progress more rapidly and may include additional features such as autonomic dysfunction and cerebellar signs.

3. Drug-Induced Parkinsonism: Some medications and drugs can cause parkinsonian symptoms, leading to a condition called drug-induced parkinsonism. It's essential to identify any potential medications that may be contributing to the symptoms.

4. Progressive Supranuclear Palsy (PSP): PSP is a rare neurodegenerative disorder with clinical similarities to Parkinson's. However, it is characterized by distinctive eye movement problems and postural instability not typically seen in Parkinson's.

5. Corticobasal Degeneration (CBD): CBD is another rare condition that can share motor symptoms with Parkinson's. It often presents with asymmetric motor dysfunction and unusual sensory symptoms.

Differential diagnosis is crucial because accurate identification of the underlying condition guides treatment and management strategies. Misdiagnosis can lead to inappropriate treatments and hinder the delivery of proper care. The expertise of a neurologist or movement disorder specialist is essential in navigating the complexities of differential diagnosis in Parkinson's and related conditions.

The Importance of Early Diagnosis in Parkinson's Disease

Early diagnosis of Parkinson's disease is of paramount importance, as it offers several significant benefits to both patients and healthcare providers. While there is no cure for Parkinson's, early identification of the disease enables timely interventions that can improve the quality of life for individuals living with the condition.

1. Initiating Treatment: Parkinson's is a progressive condition, and its symptoms tend to worsen over time. Early diagnosis allows for the prompt initiation of appropriate medical treatments, including dopaminergic medications. These drugs can help alleviate motor symptoms, improving mobility and functionality.

2. Disease Management: Early diagnosis offers a head start in developing a comprehensive management plan. This may involve a range of therapies, such as physical, occupational, and speech therapy, designed to address specific symptoms and maintain a higher level of independence.

3. Better Outcomes: Studies suggest that individuals who receive early treatment for Parkinson's disease experience improved motor function and a higher quality of life compared to those diagnosed at later stages. Early intervention can delay the progression of symptoms and complications.

4. Patient and Caregiver Education: Early diagnosis allows patients and their caregivers to proactively learn about the disease, its potential challenges, and strategies for coping. Education and support during the early stages can alleviate anxiety and enhance the patient's ability to manage the condition effectively.

5. Clinical Trials and Research: Early diagnosis provides individuals with Parkinson's the opportunity to participate in

clinical trials and research studies aimed at developing new treatments and potentially modifying the course of the disease.

In summary, early diagnosis in Parkinson's disease is a critical step in improving patient outcomes and quality of life. It empowers individuals to access the appropriate care and support, enhancing their ability to manage the condition and engage in efforts to advance our understanding and treatment of this complex neurological disorder.

CHAPTER FIVE

Treatment Options for Parkinson's Disease

Parkinson's disease is a complex condition, and its treatment aims to alleviate its hallmark motor and non-motor symptoms. The management of Parkinson's typically involves a multifaceted approach that combines medications, therapies, and lifestyle adjustments.

1. Medications: The cornerstone of Parkinson's treatment involves medications that help restore dopamine levels in the brain or mimic the action of dopamine. Levodopa is the most effective drug, often combined with carbidopa to enhance its delivery to the brain. Dopamine agonists, MAO-B inhibitors, and

anticholinergic medications are also used to manage symptoms and improve motor function.

2. Deep Brain Stimulation (DBS): For individuals with advanced Parkinson's and motor complications, deep brain stimulation is a surgical procedure that involves implanting a neurostimulator device to regulate abnormal brain activity. It can provide significant symptom relief and enhance motor control.

3. Physical Therapy: Physical therapy plays a vital role in maintaining and improving mobility, balance, and muscle strength. It can help individuals manage gait disturbances and prevent falls.

4. Occupational Therapy: Occupational therapy focuses on enhancing daily living skills, such as dressing, eating, and bathing, to maintain independence and quality of life.

5. Speech Therapy: Speech therapy is beneficial for addressing communication difficulties and swallowing problems that can accompany Parkinson's.

6. Exercise and Nutrition: Regular physical activity and a balanced diet can support overall health and minimize the progression of symptoms. Exercise can improve muscle strength, flexibility, and overall well-being.

7. Supportive Care: Non-motor symptoms, such as mood changes and cognitive impairment, often require tailored care and interventions, including counseling and medications.

Treatment for Parkinson's is highly individualized, with options and strategies tailored to the specific needs and challenges of each patient. The goal is to enhance the quality of life, maximize independence, and manage the complexities of this neurological disorder effectively. Ongoing research and developments in treatment options offer hope for better outcomes and improved care for individuals living with Parkinson's disease.

Medications: A Guide to Parkinson's Drugs

Medications play a central role in managing the symptoms of Parkinson's disease, helping individuals regain some control over their motor functions and enhance their quality of life. Understanding the different types of drugs used in the treatment of Parkinson's is essential for both patients and caregivers.

1. Levodopa (L-DOPA): Levodopa is the gold standard in Parkinson's treatment. It is converted into dopamine in the brain, helping to alleviate motor symptoms. Levodopa is often combined with carbidopa to enhance its effectiveness and minimize side effects.

2. Dopamine Agonists: These drugs mimic the action of dopamine in the brain and are often used alongside or as an alternative to levodopa. They include drugs like pramipexole and ropinirole.

3. MAO-B Inhibitors: Monoamine oxidase-B (MAO-B) inhibitors, such as selegiline and rasagiline, help increase dopamine levels by inhibiting the enzymes that break it down. They are often used in combination with levodopa.

4. Catechol-O-Methyltransferase (COMT) Inhibitors: COMT inhibitors, like entacapone and tolcapone, prolong the effects of levodopa by inhibiting the breakdown of dopamine.

5. Anticholinergic Medications: These drugs, including trihexyphenidyl and benztropine, can help control tremors and rigidity by affecting the balance of neurotransmitters in the brain.

6. Amantadine: Amantadine is used to alleviate dyskinesia, a side effect of long-term levodopa use. It can also provide some relief from motor symptoms.

Understanding the mechanisms, potential side effects, and optimal timing of these medications is crucial for a patient's overall well-being. The choice and dosages of these drugs depend on the individual's specific symptoms and progression of the disease. Regular consultations with a neurologist or movement disorder specialist are vital to ensuring the most effective and appropriate medication regimen.

Surgery and Deep Brain Stimulation in Parkinson's Disease

In cases of advanced Parkinson's disease or when medications alone no longer provide adequate symptom control, surgical interventions like Deep Brain Stimulation (DBS) can be considered. DBS is a remarkable surgical procedure that has transformed the lives of many individuals living with Parkinson's.

Deep Brain Stimulation (DBS): DBS involves the surgical implantation of a neurostimulator device, often referred to as a "brain pacemaker," into specific regions of the brain. This device delivers electrical pulses that modulate abnormal brain activity and help alleviate the motor symptoms of Parkinson's. The most commonly targeted brain areas are the subthalamic nucleus (STN) and the globus pallidus internus (GPi). DBS is particularly effective in controlling tremors, rigidity, and dyskinesia (involuntary movements), and can lead to a significant reduction in medication requirements.

Candidates for DBS: Not all individuals with Parkinson's are candidates for DBS. Typically, DBS is considered when a person has motor complications that are inadequately managed with medications, experiences disabling motor fluctuations or dyskinesia, and is mentally and physically fit for the surgery.

Benefits of DBS: DBS can significantly improve motor symptoms, enhance overall motor control, reduce medication-related side effects, and enhance the quality of life for individuals with Parkinson's. It's a reversible procedure, meaning the device can be adjusted, turned on or off, and even removed if needed.

Challenges and Considerations: DBS is a surgical procedure with potential risks and complications. Moreover, the effectiveness of DBS can vary among individuals, and it does not address non-motor symptoms of Parkinson's. Careful patient selection, ongoing evaluation, and post-operative programming are crucial for achieving the best outcomes.

Deep Brain Stimulation represents a valuable treatment option for many individuals with advanced Parkinson's, offering improved symptom control and quality of life. However, it is important for patients and their healthcare teams to carefully consider the potential benefits, risks, and individual circumstances before opting for this surgical intervention.

Complementary and Alternative Therapies in Parkinson's Disease

Complementary and alternative therapies play a supportive role in the management of Parkinson's disease, offering patients additional ways to improve their quality of life and address the multifaceted nature of the condition. These therapies are used alongside conventional medical treatments and can encompass a wide range of approaches:

1. Physical Therapy: Physical therapy can help individuals with Parkinson's improve their balance, mobility, and overall physical

function. Exercises and techniques are tailored to address specific motor symptoms and promote independence.

2. Occupational Therapy: Occupational therapy focuses on enhancing daily living skills and can help individuals with Parkinson's adapt to functional limitations. This includes strategies for dressing, cooking, and managing daily routines.

3. Speech Therapy: Speech therapy can be beneficial for individuals experiencing speech and swallowing difficulties. Techniques and exercises are aimed at improving communication and reducing the risk of aspiration.

4. Tai Chi and Yoga: Mind-body exercises like Tai Chi and Yoga can help individuals with Parkinson's improve their balance, flexibility, and overall well-being. They also provide a sense of relaxation and stress reduction.

5. Acupuncture: Acupuncture is a traditional Chinese practice that some individuals with Parkinson's have found helpful in alleviating specific symptoms like pain, stiffness, and tremors.

6. Diet and Nutrition: A balanced diet, rich in antioxidants and anti-inflammatory foods, can support overall health and potentially help manage non-motor symptoms.

7. Mindfulness and Meditation: Mindfulness and meditation techniques can assist individuals in managing stress and anxiety, which are often associated with Parkinson's.

While complementary and alternative therapies can provide valuable support, it's essential to consult with a healthcare professional, preferably one experienced in Parkinson's disease, before incorporating these practices. Safety, appropriateness, and potential interactions with prescribed medications should be carefully considered. When used in conjunction with conventional treatments and under the guidance of a healthcare team, these therapies can enhance the holistic approach to managing Parkinson's disease.

CHAPTER SIX

Living Well with Parkinson's

A diagnosis of Parkinson's disease does not mean the end of a fulfilling and meaningful life. With the right strategies and support, individuals with Parkinson's can continue to lead active and satisfying lives. Here are some key principles for living well with Parkinson's:

1. Medication Management: Consistent and accurate medication management is crucial. Work closely with your healthcare team to find the right medication regimen that effectively manages your symptoms while minimizing side effects.

2. Regular Exercise: Physical activity is essential for maintaining mobility, balance, and overall well-being. Engage in a regular

exercise routine, tailored to your abilities and preferences, which may include activities like walking, dancing, or yoga.

3. Diet and Nutrition: A balanced diet, rich in fruits, vegetables, and whole grains, can support overall health. Some studies suggest that specific diets, like the Mediterranean diet, may be beneficial for individuals with Parkinson's.

4. Mental and Emotional Well-being: Managing the emotional impact of Parkinson's is critical. Consider mindfulness, meditation, or support groups to help cope with stress, anxiety, and depression that can accompany the condition.

5. Social Engagement: Staying socially connected with family and friends is essential for emotional well-being. Don't hesitate to seek out local support groups or engage in social activities that interest you.

6. Adaptive Strategies: Find ways to adapt your living environment and daily routines to accommodate your specific needs. Occupational therapy can be particularly helpful in this regard.

7. Continued Learning: Engaging in cognitive activities and continued learning can help maintain mental sharpness. Consider reading, puzzles, or educational classes.

8. Holistic Approach: Take a holistic approach to your care, addressing both motor and non-motor symptoms. This involves regular check-ins with your healthcare team, which may include neurologists, physical therapists, and other specialists.

Living well with Parkinson's involves embracing life's challenges and opportunities, continuing to set goals, and maintaining a positive outlook. It's essential to remember that the journey with Parkinson's is unique to each individual, and ongoing support from healthcare providers, loved ones, and support networks can significantly contribute to a fulfilling life despite the condition.

Exercise and Physical Therapy in Parkinson's Disease

Exercise and physical therapy are integral components of managing Parkinson's disease, as they can help improve motor symptoms, enhance mobility, and promote overall well-being. These therapies are essential for maintaining independence and a high quality of life for individuals living with Parkinson's.

1. Improving Mobility: Exercise routines designed for Parkinson's patients focus on enhancing muscle strength, flexibility, and balance. These improvements can help counteract the motor symptoms, including bradykinesia (slowness of movement) and rigidity, making daily activities more manageable.

2. Preventing Falls: Parkinson's often leads to postural instability and an increased risk of falls. Physical therapy helps individuals learn strategies to maintain balance, reduce the likelihood of falling, and stay safe.

3. Enhancing Quality of Life: Regular exercise and physical therapy can significantly contribute to an individual's overall well-being. They help combat the sense of helplessness and inactivity that can accompany Parkinson's, providing a sense of empowerment and control.

4. Medication Management: Exercise can complement medication management by maximizing the effectiveness of certain drugs. It can also help reduce motor fluctuations, known as "off" periods, during which medication effectiveness wanes.

5. Social Engagement: Participating in group exercise classes or physical therapy sessions can provide an opportunity for social interaction and emotional support, reducing feelings of isolation that are common in Parkinson's.

6. Individualized Approach: Physical therapy is tailored to each individual's specific needs and stage of Parkinson's. A skilled therapist can design a program that addresses the unique challenges faced by the patient.

The benefits of exercise and physical therapy extend beyond symptom management; they contribute to a more fulfilling life by fostering independence, promoting social engagement, and maintaining physical and mental health. Patients with Parkinson's should consult with healthcare professionals experienced in the condition to develop a personalized exercise plan and leverage the advantages of physical therapy for improved symptom control and overall well-being.

Nutrition and Diet Recommendations for Parkinson's Disease

A well-balanced diet plays a crucial role in managing Parkinson's disease, as it can influence medication effectiveness, energy levels, and overall well-being. Here are some nutrition and diet recommendations for individuals living with Parkinson's:

1. Balanced Diet: Consume a diet rich in fruits, vegetables, whole grains, lean proteins, and healthy fats. A balanced diet provides essential nutrients and energy while supporting overall health.

2. Protein Management: Timing protein intake can be essential for optimizing the effectiveness of levodopa, a common medication for Parkinson's. Taking levodopa 30 minutes before meals or consuming lower-protein meals can help improve absorption and symptom control.

3. Hydration: Dehydration can exacerbate symptoms like constipation and blood pressure fluctuations. Staying well-hydrated is crucial for overall health.

4. Fiber-Rich Foods: A diet high in fiber can help alleviate constipation, a common non-motor symptom of Parkinson's. Include foods like whole grains, fruits, and vegetables to promote regular bowel movements.

5. Antioxidant-Rich Foods: Foods rich in antioxidants, such as berries, leafy greens, and green tea, can help combat oxidative stress, which is believed to contribute to the progression of Parkinson's.

6. Limit Processed Foods: Reducing the consumption of processed foods, high in sodium, sugar, and unhealthy fats, can help manage blood pressure and overall health.

7. Supplementation: Depending on individual needs and dietary restrictions, supplements like vitamin D, calcium, and B vitamins may be recommended.

8. Caffeine: Some studies suggest that caffeine may have a neuroprotective effect in Parkinson's disease. Moderate coffee consumption may be considered.

9. Consult a Dietitian: Working with a registered dietitian experienced in Parkinson's disease can provide tailored dietary guidance to address individual needs and challenges.

Dietary needs in Parkinson's can vary, and it's important for individuals to work with their healthcare team and a dietitian to develop a diet plan that supports their specific symptoms and overall health. A well-balanced diet can complement medical management, improve energy levels, and enhance the quality of life for those living with Parkinson's disease.

Maintaining Cognitive Health in Parkinson's Disease

Cognitive impairment is a common challenge in Parkinson's disease, and addressing cognitive health is essential for an individual's overall well-being. Here are strategies to help maintain cognitive function in the context of Parkinson's:

1. Mental Stimulation: Engage in cognitive activities that challenge the brain, such as puzzles, reading, learning a new language, or taking up a musical instrument. These activities can help keep the mind active and agile.

2. Exercise: Physical activity is not only beneficial for motor symptoms but also for cognitive health. Regular exercise can improve blood flow to the brain, promote the release of neuroprotective chemicals, and enhance cognitive function.

3. Balanced Diet: A diet rich in antioxidants, omega-3 fatty acids, and other nutrients can support brain health. These foods can

help combat oxidative stress and inflammation, which are associated with cognitive decline.

4. Sleep: Quality sleep is essential for cognitive function. Addressing sleep disturbances, such as insomnia or restless legs, can help maintain cognitive health.

5. Medication Management: Work closely with your healthcare team to ensure that Parkinson's medications are optimized for cognitive function. Some medications can impact cognitive abilities, and adjustments may be necessary.

6. Social Engagement: Staying socially active and maintaining strong social connections can stimulate cognitive function. Engage in activities that involve social interaction, such as joining support groups or participating in community events.

7. Stress Management: High levels of stress can adversely affect cognitive function. Practice stress-reduction techniques, like mindfulness or meditation, to promote mental well-being.

8. Regular Check-ups: Consistent medical follow-ups with a neurologist or movement disorder specialist can help monitor cognitive health and identify any changes or concerns.

Maintaining cognitive health is an essential aspect of living well with Parkinson's disease. While cognitive impairment can be a challenging aspect of the condition, these strategies can help individuals manage and potentially delay cognitive decline, contributing to a higher quality of life and greater independence.

CHAPTER SEVEN

Daily Strategies and Coping Mechanisms for Parkinson's Disease

Living with Parkinson's disease requires daily strategies and coping mechanisms to effectively manage symptoms, maintain quality of life, and foster a positive outlook. Here are some practical approaches for individuals with Parkinson's and their caregivers:

1. Medication Management: Consistency in taking prescribed medications at the right times is vital for symptom control. Use pill organizers, alarms, or mobile apps to help stay organized.

2. Daily Routine: Establish a structured daily routine that includes time for exercise, medication administration, meals, and relaxation. Predictable schedules can help manage symptoms and reduce stress.

3. Stay Active: Regular physical activity is crucial. Engage in exercises that focus on flexibility, strength, and balance to address motor symptoms and maintain mobility.

4. Dietary Considerations: Pay attention to when you take your medications in relation to meals to optimize their effectiveness. A dietitian can provide guidance on a balanced diet.

5. Support Groups: Join a local Parkinson's support group to connect with others who understand your experiences, share coping strategies, and provide emotional support.

6. Adaptive Devices: Use assistive devices, such as walking aids, handrails, or utensils with larger handles, to make daily tasks more manageable.

7. Mindfulness and Relaxation: Practice mindfulness and relaxation techniques to cope with stress, anxiety, and emotional challenges often associated with Parkinson's.

8. Cognitive Stimulation: Engage in mental activities like puzzles, games, and hobbies that stimulate cognitive function.

9. Communication: Effective communication is vital. Inform your healthcare team about any changes or concerns, and maintain open and honest communication with family and friends.

10. Caregiver Support: Caregivers also need support. Reach out to caregiver support networks, and don't hesitate to ask for help when needed.

Coping with Parkinson's is a journey that requires flexibility, adaptability, and a proactive approach. By incorporating these daily strategies and coping mechanisms, individuals with Parkinson's can enhance their overall well-being, maintain independence, and lead fulfilling lives despite the challenges posed by the condition.

Managing Motor Symptoms in Parkinson's Disease

Motor symptoms, including tremors, bradykinesia (slowness of movement), muscle rigidity, and postural instability, are the hallmark features of Parkinson's disease. Effective management of these symptoms is essential for improving mobility, function, and overall quality of life. Here are strategies to help manage motor symptoms:

1. Medication Management: The primary approach to managing motor symptoms in Parkinson's is medication. Levodopa, dopamine agonists, and other drugs are prescribed to alleviate symptoms and enhance mobility. Close collaboration with a neurologist is crucial to find the most suitable medication regimen.

2. Timely Medication: Take medications as prescribed, adhering to a strict schedule. Some individuals may benefit from extended-release formulations to maintain a consistent level of medication in the body.

3. Dietary Considerations: Pay attention to protein intake, as it can affect the absorption of levodopa. Coordinate the timing of meals and medication to optimize drug effectiveness.

4. Physical Therapy: Regular physical therapy helps improve muscle strength, flexibility, and balance. Specific exercises can target motor symptoms, enhancing mobility and posture.

5. Occupational Therapy: Occupational therapists can provide strategies for adapting daily activities to overcome motor challenges, such as dressing, eating, and bathing.

6. Deep Brain Stimulation (DBS): For individuals with advanced motor complications, DBS can be considered as a surgical option to help control symptoms, especially when medications alone are no longer effective.

7. Lifestyle Adjustments: Adjust your living environment and daily routines to accommodate motor limitations. Use assistive devices or home modifications when needed.

8. Regular Exercise: Engage in regular physical activity to maintain muscle tone, flexibility, and overall physical well-being. Activities like walking, cycling, and dancing can be beneficial.

Effective management of motor symptoms requires a comprehensive approach that combines medication, therapy, and lifestyle adjustments. Regular follow-ups with healthcare professionals are essential to fine-tune the treatment plan, ensuring the best possible symptom control and quality of life for individuals living with Parkinson's disease.

Strategies for Dealing with Non-Motor Symptoms in Parkinson's Disease

Parkinson's disease is not limited to motor symptoms; it also frequently presents a range of non-motor symptoms that can significantly impact a person's quality of life. Coping with these non-motor symptoms requires a multifaceted approach. Here are some strategies to help manage non-motor aspects of the condition:

1. Communication: Open and honest communication with healthcare providers is essential. Discuss any non-motor symptoms, such as mood changes, sleep disturbances, or cognitive challenges, to ensure they are addressed appropriately.

2. Medication Review: Some non-motor symptoms can be influenced by Parkinson's medications. Periodic medication reviews can help adjust dosages or switch medications to manage these symptoms better.

3. Sleep Hygiene: Practicing good sleep hygiene, such as maintaining a consistent sleep schedule and creating a comfortable sleeping environment, can help alleviate sleep disturbances.

4. Mental Health Support: Seek psychological support, counseling, or therapy to address mood changes, anxiety, and depression. Social engagement and support groups can also provide emotional support.

5. Physical Activity: Regular exercise has been shown to improve mood and reduce anxiety and depression. Engage in physical activities tailored to your abilities and interests.

6. Cognitive Stimulation: Mental exercises, puzzles, and cognitive activities can help maintain cognitive function and manage memory and thinking difficulties.

7. Diet and Nutrition: A balanced diet and proper hydration can support overall well-being and may help manage non-motor symptoms like constipation and fatigue.

8. Stress Reduction: Stress management techniques such as mindfulness, meditation, or relaxation exercises can help cope with emotional challenges and enhance mental well-being.

9. Medication for Specific Symptoms: Some non-motor symptoms, like hallucinations, may require targeted medication management. Discuss these symptoms with your healthcare provider to explore potential treatments.

Coping with non-motor symptoms in Parkinson's requires a holistic approach that encompasses physical, emotional, and mental well-being. The key is individualized care that addresses specific challenges, improves quality of life, and empowers individuals with Parkinson's to continue leading fulfilling lives despite these non-motor aspects of the condition.

Caregiving and Support in Parkinson's Disease

Caregivers play an essential role in supporting individuals living with Parkinson's disease. Their dedication and assistance can significantly improve the quality of life for both patients and caregivers themselves. Here are key considerations for caregiving and support in Parkinson's:

1. Education: Caregivers should strive to educate themselves about Parkinson's disease. Understanding its symptoms, progression, and treatment options can help them provide better care and support.

2. Communication: Open and honest communication between caregivers and individuals with Parkinson's is essential. It allows for discussing concerns, needs, and potential changes in care strategies.

3. Medication Management: Caregivers can assist in ensuring that individuals with Parkinson's take their medications as prescribed and at the right times. Monitoring medication schedules and effectiveness is critical.

4. Mobility and Daily Living Assistance: Parkinson's can impact mobility and daily living tasks. Caregivers may need to assist with activities like dressing, grooming, and meal preparation as symptoms progress.

5. Emotional Support: Caregivers should be attuned to the emotional challenges that can arise with Parkinson's, including mood changes, anxiety, and depression. Providing emotional support, understanding, and empathy is crucial.

6. Physical Therapy: Encouraging and supporting individuals with Parkinson's in engaging in physical therapy exercises can help maintain mobility and improve motor function.

7. Respite Care: Caregivers should consider their own well-being and seek respite care when needed to prevent caregiver burnout and maintain their own health.

8. Support Groups: Both individuals with Parkinson's and their caregivers can benefit from participating in support groups. These groups offer a sense of community, shared experiences, and practical advice.

9. Regular Check-ups: Staying informed about medical appointments and accompanying individuals with Parkinson's to consultations ensures that their care remains comprehensive and up to date.

10. Adaptive Strategies: As symptoms evolve, caregivers can work with healthcare professionals and occupational therapists to learn adaptive strategies for coping with challenges in daily life.

Caregiving in Parkinson's can be challenging, but it is also deeply rewarding. It requires patience, compassion, and a proactive approach to ensuring that individuals with Parkinson's have the best possible support to lead fulfilling lives despite the condition. Caregivers themselves should not underestimate the importance of self-care and seeking their own support to continue providing the best care possible.

CHAPTER EIGHT

A Journey of Hope: Personal Stories in Parkinson's Disease

Personal stories of individuals living with Parkinson's disease and their caregivers offer a powerful and inspirational perspective on the challenges and triumphs in the face of this condition. These narratives serve as beacons of hope and resilience, demonstrating that life with Parkinson's can still be a meaningful and fulfilling journey.

These stories often revolve around the themes of courage, determination, and unwavering support. They showcase the incredible strength it takes to face the daily battles that Parkinson's presents, from motor and non-motor symptoms to emotional and cognitive challenges.

In these personal accounts, individuals often share how they've adapted to their changing circumstances, embracing innovative treatments, and learning to manage symptoms effectively. They emphasize the importance of a positive mindset and the vital role of support networks, from healthcare professionals to family and friends.

These stories also highlight the sense of empowerment that can come from sharing experiences, from participating in support groups to becoming advocates for Parkinson's awareness and research. They remind us that despite the adversities, there is hope, and there is a path to living well with Parkinson's disease. These narratives offer valuable insights and inspiration to those newly diagnosed with Parkinson's, their families, and caregivers. They remind us that, even in the face of a challenging diagnosis, life can be full of purpose, joy, and meaningful connections.

Real-life Accounts from People Living with Parkinson's

Real-life accounts from individuals living with Parkinson's disease provide a deeply personal and honest look into the everyday challenges, triumphs, and resilience that characterize their journey. These accounts humanize the condition, breaking down stereotypes and fostering understanding. They offer several key insights:

1. Variability of Symptoms: These accounts reveal the immense variability in how Parkinson's manifests. Each person's experience is unique, with a diverse range of motor and non-motor symptoms.

2. Emotional and Psychological Impact: Personal stories shed light on the emotional and psychological impact of Parkinson's, including feelings of frustration, isolation, and courage in facing adversity.

3. Family and Caregiver Dynamics: Real-life accounts often touch on the invaluable support of family and caregivers, highlighting the vital role they play in helping individuals manage the condition.

4. Adaptive Strategies: Individuals with Parkinson's share their creative adaptive strategies, which can serve as inspiration for others. These include finding new hobbies, participating in support groups, and advocating for awareness and research.

5. Hope and Resilience: Despite the challenges, these accounts often emphasize the strength, resilience, and hope that people with Parkinson's embody. They inspire others to confront their own struggles with determination and optimism.

6. Advocacy and Awareness: Many individuals living with Parkinson's become advocates for awareness and research, using their stories to drive change and improve the lives of others facing the condition.

Real-life accounts are not only a source of inspiration but also a means of reducing stigma and encouraging empathy. They show that life with Parkinson's, while challenging, can be meaningful and full of hope, reminding everyone that, even in the face of adversity, there is strength, determination, and the potential for a fulfilling life.

Insights from Caregivers and Family Members in Parkinson's Care

Caregivers and family members of individuals living with Parkinson's disease offer invaluable insights into the journey of care and support. Their experiences illuminate the challenges, triumphs, and dedication required to help a loved one navigate life with Parkinson's. Here are some key insights:

1. Empathy and Understanding: Caregivers and family members often gain a profound understanding of the physical and emotional struggles faced by individuals with Parkinson's. This empathy fosters strong bonds and compassion.

2. Adaptive Resilience: These caregivers demonstrate remarkable adaptive resilience. They learn to cope with the

evolving nature of the condition, adjusting their support and routines to address changing needs.

3. Advocacy and Education: Many family members become advocates for Parkinson's awareness and research. They actively seek knowledge, engage in support groups, and collaborate with healthcare professionals to ensure their loved one receives the best care.

4. Balancing Self-care: Caring for someone with Parkinson's can be demanding, and family members often emphasize the importance of self-care. They recognize that taking care of themselves is vital to provide effective support.

5. Unconditional Love: The unwavering commitment of caregivers and family members shines through. Their dedication and love play a pivotal role in helping individuals with Parkinson's maintain their independence and quality of life.

6. Emotional Support: Caregivers and family members provide emotional support that is a vital lifeline for those with Parkinson's. They create a safe and understanding space for

open communication about the challenges and emotional aspects of the condition.

7. Respect and Dignity: These insights emphasize the importance of treating individuals with Parkinson's with respect and preserving their dignity, even when caregiving tasks involve personal care.

The experiences of caregivers and family members reflect the power of love, resilience, and the importance of building a strong support network. Their insights inspire empathy and appreciation for the vital role they play in enhancing the quality of life for individuals with Parkinson's disease.

CHAPTER NINE

Research and Future Prospects in Parkinson's Disease

Ongoing research in Parkinson's disease holds promise for advancements in understanding, treatment, and ultimately finding a cure for this complex neurological condition. Here are key areas of research and future prospects:

1. Genetics: The role of genetics in Parkinson's is a growing area of focus. Identifying genetic markers associated with the condition can help in early detection and personalized treatment approaches.

2. Neuroprotection: Researchers are actively exploring methods to protect and preserve dopamine-producing neurons in the brain. These approaches aim to slow down or halt disease progression.

3. Stem Cell Therapy: Stem cell research offers the potential to replace damaged neurons in the brain, providing a regenerative approach to Parkinson's treatment.

4. Deep Brain Stimulation (DBS): Ongoing studies seek to optimize DBS techniques, develop new brain targets, and improve outcomes for individuals with advanced Parkinson's.

5. Non-Motor Symptoms: There is a growing understanding of non-motor symptoms, and research aims to improve the diagnosis and management of these often-overlooked aspects of the disease.

6. Biomarker Discovery: Identifying reliable biomarkers for Parkinson's can aid in early diagnosis, tracking disease progression, and evaluating treatment effectiveness.

7. Drug Development: Ongoing drug development research focuses on refining existing medications, exploring novel treatment options, and reducing side effects.

8. Patient-Centered Care: Research emphasizes the importance of patient-centered care, tailored to individual needs and

preferences, enhancing the quality of life for people living with Parkinson's.

The future holds great potential for innovative treatments, improved symptom management, and a deeper understanding of the underlying causes of Parkinson's disease. As researchers continue to explore these areas, they bring hope for better care, increased quality of life, and, ultimately, a cure for Parkinson's disease. This collective effort brings optimism for the many individuals and families affected by this condition.

Breakthroughs and Promising Research in Parkinson's Disease

Over the years, groundbreaking research and discoveries have offered hope and potential new avenues for the management and treatment of Parkinson's disease. Here are some notable breakthroughs and promising research areas:

1. Alpha-Synuclein: Researchers are making strides in understanding alpha-synuclein, a protein associated with Parkinson's. This understanding opens doors to targeted therapies that aim to reduce the accumulation of toxic alpha-synuclein clumps in the brain.

2. Gene Therapy: Gene therapy approaches are being explored to modify genes associated with Parkinson's, potentially offering disease-modifying treatments.

3. Immunotherapies: Immunotherapies designed to harness the body's immune system to target and clear abnormal proteins implicated in Parkinson's are under investigation.

4. Neuroinflammation: Research into neuroinflammation's role in Parkinson's is providing insights into potential anti-inflammatory treatments that may slow disease progression.

5. Repurposed Drugs: Existing drugs used for other conditions are being repurposed and tested for their potential in treating Parkinson's.

6. Regenerative Medicine: Stem cell therapies hold promise for replacing damaged dopamine-producing neurons in the brain, potentially restoring lost motor function.

7. Telemedicine and Wearable Technologies: Advancements in telemedicine and wearable technologies are facilitating remote monitoring and early intervention, improving patient care and data collection for research.

While these breakthroughs and ongoing research provide optimism, it's important to acknowledge that finding a cure or fully effective treatments for Parkinson's is a complex and ongoing process. Collaborative efforts among researchers, healthcare providers, individuals living with Parkinson's, and their families are vital in advancing our understanding and improving the lives of those affected by this condition.

Clinical Trials and Emerging Treatments in Parkinson's Disease

Clinical trials are at the forefront of Parkinson's disease research, offering a pathway to test and refine emerging treatments. These trials are essential for developing new therapies and improving the lives of individuals living with the condition. Here are some insights into the significance of clinical trials and the emerging treatments they explore:

1. Disease Modification: Clinical trials are focused on developing disease-modifying treatments that can slow or halt the progression of Parkinson's, which could transform the way the condition is managed.

2. Symptom Management: Emerging treatments aim to address not only motor symptoms but also non-motor symptoms, improving overall quality of life.

3. Personalized Medicine: Ongoing research is exploring the concept of personalized medicine, tailoring treatments to an individual's unique genetic and biological profile.

4. Neuroprotection: Many trials investigate treatments designed to protect and preserve dopamine-producing neurons, delaying the loss of motor function.

5. Immunotherapies: Immunotherapies, which harness the immune system to target abnormal proteins associated with Parkinson's, are a promising avenue.

6. Alpha-Synuclein Therapies: Treatments targeting alpha-synuclein aggregation are in development, offering potential solutions to the protein's role in the disease.

7. Wearable Technologies: Clinical trials often incorporate wearable devices and digital health platforms to monitor symptoms and treatment effectiveness.

It's important for individuals with Parkinson's and their families to consider participating in clinical trials, as they offer access to cutting-edge treatments and contribute to the advancement of our understanding of the disease. Through participation, individuals can be at the forefront of innovation, and their experiences can help shape the future of Parkinson's care. Clinical trials play a vital role in bringing hope and progress to those affected by this condition.

The Quest for a Cure in Parkinson's Disease

The quest for a cure for Parkinson's disease is a relentless journey driven by a global community of researchers, healthcare professionals, individuals living with the condition, and their families. This collective effort is marked by unwavering dedication and collaboration to find a definitive solution for this complex neurodegenerative disorder.

Several key elements define the ongoing quest for a cure:

1. Interdisciplinary Collaboration: Scientists, clinicians, and healthcare professionals from various fields collaborate to

advance our understanding of Parkinson's, creating a multidisciplinary approach to research.

2. Patient-Centered Focus: Individuals living with Parkinson's are at the heart of research efforts, with their experiences, challenges, and insights guiding investigations into treatments and interventions.

3. Translational Research: Studies bridge the gap between laboratory discoveries and real-world applications, seeking to translate promising findings into practical treatments.

4. Global Initiatives: International collaborations and initiatives bring together the brightest minds and the most extensive resources to tackle Parkinson's on a global scale.

5. Advocacy and Awareness: Patient advocacy groups and organizations play a crucial role in raising awareness, funding research, and supporting the drive for a cure.

6. Innovation and Technology: Emerging technologies and innovative approaches, such as genetics, stem cells, and

precision medicine, offer new pathways for developing treatments and ultimately finding a cure.

The quest for a cure is a long and challenging journey, but it is fueled by hope, determination, and the belief that one day, Parkinson's will be conquered. Until then, the collaborative efforts of the global community continue to drive progress and inspire optimism for a future without Parkinson's disease.

CHAPTER TEN

Resources and Support for Parkinson's Disease

Navigating life with Parkinson's disease can be challenging, but a wealth of resources and support is available to help individuals and their families face these challenges with confidence. Here are some key sources of assistance and guidance:

1. Parkinson's Organizations: Numerous national and international organizations, such as the Michael J. Fox Foundation, the Parkinson's Foundation, and local Parkinson's associations, offer a wealth of information, support groups, educational materials, and advocacy efforts.

2. Healthcare Professionals: Neurologists, movement disorder specialists, physical therapists, and occupational therapists play crucial roles in managing Parkinson's. They provide medical guidance and therapies to enhance quality of life.

3. Caregiver Support Groups: Caregiver support groups offer a sense of community, emotional support, and practical advice for those supporting loved ones with Parkinson's.

4. Patient Support Groups: Local and online support groups bring together individuals living with Parkinson's to share experiences, strategies, and coping mechanisms.

5. Educational Materials: Access to literature, webinars, and informational resources helps individuals and caregivers gain a deeper understanding of Parkinson's and its management.

6. Telemedicine: Remote healthcare services have become more prevalent, allowing individuals to consult with specialists and access care from the comfort of their homes.

7. Legal and Financial Assistance: Legal professionals can help individuals plan for future care needs, while financial advisors can assist in managing the cost of treatment.

8. Community Services: Local community services, such as home healthcare, meal delivery, and transportation assistance, can make daily life more manageable.

9. Research Participation: Enrolling in clinical trials and studies not only contributes to Parkinson's research but also provides access to cutting-edge treatments and therapies.

10.

The comprehensive network of resources and support available for Parkinson's empowers individuals to lead fulfilling lives, maintain independence, and face the condition with resilience and hope. These resources and support systems ensure that no one has to face Parkinson's alone.

Parkinson's Organizations and Support Groups: Empowering Communities

Parkinson's disease organizations and support groups play a pivotal role in empowering individuals living with the condition and their families. These dedicated entities offer a broad range of resources and support, fostering a sense of community, advocacy, and education. Here's a closer look at their significance:

1. Information and Education: Parkinson's organizations provide a wealth of information about the condition, its symptoms, and the latest research. They offer educational materials, webinars, and expert advice to help individuals and families gain a deeper understanding of Parkinson's.

2. Support Networks: Support groups, often organized by these organizations, connect individuals living with Parkinson's and caregivers. These groups provide a safe space to share

experiences, insights, and emotional support, reducing feelings of isolation.

3. Advocacy: Many Parkinson's organizations advocate for improved healthcare policies, research funding, and public awareness. They work tirelessly to represent the interests of the Parkinson's community at local, national, and international levels.

4. Clinical Trials: These organizations often facilitate access to clinical trials and studies, allowing individuals to participate in cutting-edge research and potentially gain access to new treatments.

5. Community Engagement: Through local chapters and events, Parkinson's organizations foster a sense of community and engagement, connecting people facing similar challenges.

6. Professional Networks: These organizations collaborate with healthcare professionals, including neurologists and therapists, to ensure individuals with Parkinson's receive the best possible care and support.

7. Financial Assistance: Some organizations offer financial assistance and resources to help individuals and families manage the cost of treatment and care.

The combined efforts of Parkinson's organizations and support groups create a lifeline for those affected by the condition. They promote a sense of empowerment, reduce stigma, and provide essential tools for navigating the challenges associated with Parkinson's disease. By bringing together communities, raising awareness, and advocating for research, these organizations are instrumental in improving the quality of life for individuals living with Parkinson's.

Online Resources and Communities in Parkinson's Care

The digital age has revolutionized access to information and support for individuals living with Parkinson's disease and their caregivers. Online resources and communities have become invaluable tools in navigating the complexities of this condition. Here's how they play a crucial role:

1. Information and Education: Websites, forums, and educational platforms provide an abundance of information about Parkinson's disease, its symptoms, treatment options, and research developments. This readily accessible knowledge empowers individuals to make informed decisions about their care.

2. Support Groups: Online support groups and communities offer a sense of belonging and understanding. They connect people facing similar challenges, allowing them to share experiences, advice, and emotional support, even across vast distances.

3. Telemedicine: Telehealth services enable remote consultations with healthcare professionals. This technology expands access to medical care, making it more convenient for individuals living with Parkinson's.

4. Advocacy and Awareness: Online communities serve as platforms for advocacy, raising awareness, and lobbying for

improved healthcare policies and research funding to benefit the Parkinson's community.

5. Clinical Trial Information: Websites and databases provide up-to-date information about clinical trials and research studies, helping individuals connect with opportunities for participating in cutting-edge research.

6. Caregiver Resources: Online platforms offer resources and support for caregivers, equipping them with information, strategies, and networks to provide better care.

7. Patient Blogs and Personal Stories: Many individuals with Parkinson's share their personal journeys and insights through blogs and social media, offering encouragement and inspiration to others.

These online resources and communities have become lifelines for those affected by Parkinson's, enhancing access to knowledge, support, and connectivity. They exemplify the power of technology in reducing isolation, increasing awareness, and ultimately improving the quality of life for individuals living with this condition.

Tips for Navigating Healthcare Systems with Parkinson's Disease

Navigating the healthcare system with Parkinson's disease can be a complex process, but with the right approach, individuals and their caregivers can optimize their care and ensure their needs are met. Here are some valuable tips for navigating the healthcare system effectively:

1. Build a Knowledge Base: Educate yourself about Parkinson's disease, its symptoms, and treatment options. Understanding the condition empowers you to make informed decisions about your care.

2. Create a Care Team: Assemble a multidisciplinary care team that includes a neurologist, movement disorder specialist, physical therapist, and other specialists as needed. Collaborate with healthcare professionals who are experienced in managing Parkinson's.

3. Keep Detailed Records: Maintain a comprehensive record of your medical history, medications, and symptom changes. This information is invaluable for healthcare providers in tailoring your treatment plan.

4. Open Communication: Foster open and honest communication with your care team. Discuss your symptoms, concerns, and goals to ensure your care plan aligns with your needs.

5. Stay Informed: Stay up to date on the latest research, treatments, and clinical trials related to Parkinson's disease. Knowledge is a powerful tool in advocating for your care.

6. Access Support Groups: Join local or online support groups for individuals with Parkinson's. These communities provide a valuable network of shared experiences and advice.

7. Consider Telemedicine: Explore telehealth options for medical consultations, as they can offer convenience, particularly for follow-up visits.

8. Advocate for Yourself: Don't hesitate to advocate for the care you need. If you feel that your needs are not being met, speak up and seek second opinions if necessary.

9. Plan for Future Care: Consider long-term care planning, including advanced directives, legal matters, and financial arrangements.

10. Review Insurance Coverage: Understand your insurance coverage and be aware of any changes in your plan. This ensures you can access the necessary services without unexpected financial burdens.

Navigating the healthcare system with Parkinson's disease requires active involvement and advocacy. By following these tips and seeking the support of healthcare professionals and support networks, individuals and their caregivers can enhance their quality of care and overall well-being.

CHAPTER ELEVEN

A Vision for a Parkinson's-Friendly World

In envisioning a Parkinson's-friendly world, we aspire to create an environment that embraces compassion, understanding, and empowerment for all individuals affected by this neurodegenerative condition. This vision encompasses several essential elements:

1. Awareness and Education: A Parkinson's-friendly world is one where awareness is widespread and understanding of the condition is common. Education about the disease's symptoms, challenges, and impact promotes empathy and reduces stigma.

2. Inclusive Healthcare: Healthcare systems are accessible, patient-centered, and equipped to provide comprehensive care tailored to the unique needs of individuals living with Parkinson's.

3. Advancements in Research: A world that prioritizes Parkinson's is one where research thrives. Breakthroughs in treatment, diagnostics, and ultimately a cure are supported and celebrated.

4. Community Support: Local and global communities actively engage in support networks and advocacy efforts, offering a sense of belonging and empowerment to those affected by Parkinson's.

5. Quality of Life: The focus is on enhancing the quality of life for individuals with Parkinson's. This includes improved symptom management, emotional support, and opportunities for meaningful participation in daily life.

6. Inclusivity and Accessibility: A Parkinson's-friendly world considers the needs of those with mobility limitations and other

challenges, making public spaces, transportation, and infrastructure accessible to all.

7. Reduced Stigma: The world we envision is one where stereotypes and misunderstandings about Parkinson's are replaced with compassion, acceptance, and encouragement.

8. Global Collaboration: International cooperation, research partnerships, and shared knowledge pave the way for more effective treatments and therapies.

This vision for a Parkinson's-friendly world is not only attainable but essential. It requires collective efforts from individuals, communities, healthcare systems, and governments. By working together, we can create a world where people living with Parkinson's are supported, understood, and empowered to live their lives to the fullest, regardless of the challenges they face.

Advocacy and Raising Awareness for Parkinson's Disease

Advocacy and raising awareness play a vital role in improving the lives of individuals living with Parkinson's disease. Here's how these efforts create positive change:

1. Reducing Stigma: Advocacy and awareness campaigns challenge misconceptions and stereotypes about Parkinson's, fostering understanding and empathy. This reduces the stigma associated with the condition.

2. Increased Research Funding: Advocacy efforts aim to secure more funding for Parkinson's research, driving advancements in treatment, care, and ultimately a cure.

3. Policy and Legislation: Advocacy can lead to the development of policies and legislation that prioritize the needs of individuals with Parkinson's, such as accessible healthcare and support services.

4. Patient-Centered Care: By advocating for patient-centered care, individuals with Parkinson's gain a stronger voice in their treatment and better access to tailored support.

5. Support Networks: Raising awareness creates opportunities for individuals and their families to connect with support networks, strengthening their ability to navigate the challenges of the condition.

6. Early Diagnosis: Awareness campaigns can encourage early diagnosis and intervention, leading to more effective symptom management and improved quality of life.

7. Research Participation: By raising awareness of clinical trials and research opportunities, more individuals are likely to participate, accelerating scientific progress.

8. Global Collaborations: Advocacy efforts foster international collaboration in the fight against Parkinson's, bringing together experts, researchers, and resources from around the world.

9. Community Engagement: Raising awareness encourages community involvement and support for those affected by Parkinson's, promoting a sense of unity and shared purpose.

Advocacy and awareness initiatives are instrumental in creating a world that is more compassionate, knowledgeable, and supportive of individuals with Parkinson's disease. By elevating the voices and experiences of those affected, we work toward a brighter future with improved care, treatment options, and ultimately, a cure.

Breaking Down Stigma: Redefining Parkinson's Disease

Breaking down stigma associated with Parkinson's disease is essential to creating a more inclusive and empathetic world for individuals affected by this condition. Here's how we can work to redefine perceptions and challenge stigmatizing beliefs:

1. Education: Education is a powerful tool in dismantling stigma. By increasing awareness about Parkinson's disease, its symptoms, and the challenges individuals face, we can replace ignorance with understanding.

2. Personal Stories: Sharing personal stories of individuals living with Parkinson's and their caregivers humanizes the condition. It highlights their courage and resilience, dispelling stereotypes.

3. Language Matters: Use inclusive and respectful language when discussing Parkinson's. Avoid derogatory terms or casual jokes that perpetuate stigmatizing beliefs.

4. Media Representation: Advocate for accurate and sensitive portrayals of Parkinson's in the media to challenge stereotypes and raise awareness.

5. Community Engagement: Engage with the Parkinson's community, attend events, and participate in support groups to connect with individuals and challenge your own preconceptions.

6. Advocacy: Support advocacy efforts that aim to reduce stigma and improve the lives of those with Parkinson's. Lobby for

research funding, accessible healthcare, and public policies that prioritize the needs of individuals with the condition.

7. Empathy and Support: Offer empathy and support to those living with Parkinson's and their caregivers. Simple acts of kindness can go a long way in reducing stigma.

8. Normalize Conversations: Encourage open and honest conversations about Parkinson's, so individuals feel comfortable sharing their experiences and seeking help when needed.

Breaking down the stigma surrounding Parkinson's disease creates a more compassionate and inclusive society where individuals living with the condition can thrive without fear of judgment or discrimination. It begins with education, empathy, and a commitment to challenge stigmatizing beliefs.

Promoting a Supportive Society for Parkinson's Disease

Promoting a supportive society for Parkinson's disease is a collective effort that fosters understanding, compassion, and inclusivity for individuals and families affected by this condition. Here's how we can work together to create a more supportive environment:

1. Raise Awareness: Increased awareness about Parkinson's disease is the first step in building a supportive society. Educate the public about the condition, its challenges, and the experiences of those living with it.

2. Reduce Stigma: Challenge stereotypes and stigmatizing beliefs associated with Parkinson's. Encourage empathy and understanding to create a more accepting society.

3. Accessible Healthcare: Advocate for healthcare systems that are accessible, affordable, and patient-centered. This ensures

that individuals with Parkinson's can easily access the care and resources they need.

4. Community Involvement: Engage with local and national Parkinson's organizations and support groups. Participate in events, share experiences, and offer your support to those facing the condition.

5. Inclusive Design: Promote the design of public spaces, transportation, and infrastructure that accommodates the needs of individuals with mobility limitations and other challenges associated with Parkinson's.

6. Empower Individuals: Encourage individuals with Parkinson's to be active participants in their care and advocate for their needs. Empower them to have a voice in their treatment plans.

7. Advocacy: Support advocacy efforts that aim to secure research funding, improved healthcare policies, and better access to treatment for Parkinson's disease.

8. Volunteer and Donate: Contribute your time or resources to Parkinson's organizations and initiatives, helping to advance research, patient support, and awareness.

A supportive society for Parkinson's recognizes the worth and dignity of every individual, irrespective of their condition. By promoting understanding, reducing stigma, and advocating for better care and research, we can create an environment where individuals with Parkinson's can lead fulfilling and meaningful lives.

CHAPTER TWELVE

Empowering Yourself and Loved Ones in the Face of Parkinson's Disease

Empowerment is a vital component of the journey with Parkinson's disease. Here are some ways to empower yourself and your loved ones in the face of this condition:

1. Education: Knowledge is power. Educate yourself about Parkinson's disease, its symptoms, treatments, and available resources. Understanding the condition is the first step in taking control of your health.

2. Effective Communication: Encourage open and honest communication with healthcare professionals. Discuss your concerns, goals, and treatment options to make informed decisions.

3. Advocacy: Be your own advocate. Take an active role in your healthcare, ask questions, and express your needs and preferences. Advocate for better care and increased awareness of Parkinson's.

4. Support Networks: Build a strong support system. Connect with support groups and organizations that provide emotional, informational, and practical assistance for both individuals with Parkinson's and their caregivers.

5. Healthy Lifestyle: Embrace a healthy lifestyle by maintaining a balanced diet, engaging in regular physical activity, and managing stress. These habits can have a positive impact on your well-being.

6. Goal Setting: Set achievable goals to maintain a sense of purpose and motivation. Whether it's maintaining independence or pursuing a specific hobby, having goals can empower you.

7. Research Participation: Consider participating in clinical trials or studies to contribute to the advancement of Parkinson's research. Your involvement can make a meaningful difference.

8. Resilience: Cultivate resilience and a positive mindset. While Parkinson's presents challenges, a resilient attitude can help you face them with strength and determination.

9. Family and Caregiver Engagement: Involve your loved ones in the journey, ensuring they understand the condition and feel equipped to provide support.

Empowerment is about taking control of your life and actively participating in your care. By staying informed, advocating for your needs, and building a strong support network, you can enhance your quality of life and that of your loved ones as you navigate Parkinson's disease together.

Embracing Life with Parkinson's: Finding Meaning and Joy

While Parkinson's disease brings its challenges, it is possible to live a fulfilling and meaningful life. Embracing life with Parkinson's involves a positive mindset, resilience, and a focus on what brings joy and purpose. Here are some key principles to consider:

1. Acceptance: Accepting the diagnosis is the first step in embracing life with Parkinson's. Acknowledge the condition and its challenges, but don't let it define your entire identity.

2. Lifestyle Choices: Maintain a healthy lifestyle by engaging in regular physical activity, following a balanced diet, and managing stress. These choices can have a positive impact on your well-being.

3. Mindfulness and Coping: Practice mindfulness and develop coping strategies to deal with symptoms and emotional

challenges. Mindfulness can help you stay present and find peace in the moment.

4. Setting Goals: Set achievable goals that reflect your interests and passions. Whether it's pursuing a hobby, traveling, or spending quality time with loved ones, having goals can give your life purpose.

5. Support Network: Build a support network of friends, family, and support groups who understand your journey and offer emotional support.

6. Advocacy: Advocate for yourself and others living with Parkinson's. Get involved in raising awareness and fighting for better care and research funding.

7. Adaptive Living: Adapt your living environment to suit your needs. This might involve making your home more accessible or using assistive devices.

8. Creative Outlets: Explore creative outlets like art, music, or writing as a way to express your emotions and find joy in self-expression.

9. Sharing Your Story: Sharing your experience with Parkinson's can not only inspire others but also create a sense of purpose for yourself.

Embracing life with Parkinson's means focusing on what you can do and what brings you happiness. It's about finding strength in resilience and cherishing the moments that make life meaningful. With the right mindset and support, you can continue to live a fulfilling and joyous life.

A Message of Hope in the Face of Parkinson's Disease

In the midst of the challenges posed by Parkinson's disease, a message of hope shines through. Hope is a powerful force that can inspire individuals and their loved ones to persevere, adapt, and find joy in life. Here is a message of hope for those on the journey with Parkinson's:

Parkinson's disease may bring uncertainty and change, but it does not define who you are. Your strength, resilience, and the love and support of your family and community are sources of boundless hope. You are not alone on this journey; millions of individuals around the world are navigating it with you.

Hope resides in the ongoing research and advancements in understanding Parkinson's. Every day, scientists and healthcare professionals work tirelessly to improve treatments, uncover new therapies, and ultimately find a cure. Your involvement in research and clinical trials contributes to these efforts.

Every moment you embrace life with Parkinson's is a testament to your courage and determination. It's a reminder that despite the challenges, there is joy to be found, purpose to be fulfilled, and a life well-lived.

So, let hope be your guide. With hope, there is strength. With hope, there is progress. With hope, there is the promise of a brighter future. Parkinson's may be a part of your journey, but it does not have to be the entirety of it. Embrace life with hope, for it is a beacon that lights your path towards a more fulfilling and joyful tomorrow.